Stronger Than Lyme

My Battle and Blueprint for
Overcoming This Strange Disease

Jen Deering

Table of Contents

BE PARANOID

Before I begin my story, please allow me to offer the best advice I believe I can. Be paranoid.

Paranoid is a strong word, but not unjustly used in relation to Lyme disease. The key to having the best possible outcome should you contract Lyme disease is early detection and treatment. The less time the bacteria that causes Lyme disease, *Borrelia burgdorferi*, get to implant and live in your body, the less short-term and possible long-term damage the infection will cause.

Lyme disease is frequently called the great impostor because the infection mimics a variety of common aliments across the population. For example, common symptoms could be fatigue, general aches and pains, flu-like symptoms, headache, or absentmindedness. In addition to symptoms mimicking common ailments in the early stages of infection, symptom presentation is not consistent within one individual. Meaning, one may notice they have achy knees one week, and a week or so later they may have flu like symptoms and or heavy fatigue. At first blush, neither of these issues seem like a big deal, and certainly don't seem related. The tricky nature of the disease and its enigmatic early presentation is exactly what makes it worrisome. An individual may not realize anything is even wrong, until something is REALLY wrong.

The bacteria that cause Lyme disease seem to have a strong drive to live and are adept at hiding in plain sight. Lyme disease is a sly bastard, but the good news is, especially here in the Northeast, that we're getting better at catching it early. Prompt treatment of Lyme reduces the disease to virtually a non-issue and essentially mitigates all risk of long-term or chronic effects of the disease.

Still, many cases slide by, and there is a large contingent of residents in, or at least from the Northeast, who got infected years ago and experience lingering symptoms of Lyme. The CDC's latest statistics show that 60% of Lyme disease patients report ongoing symptoms. This is exactly why a healthy dose of paranoia is good. Prompt detection of Lyme is extremely beneficial.

There isn't a single aspect of contracting Lyme disease that makes timely detection easy. Lyme disease is transmitted to humans through a bite from a tiny parasitic tick, *Ixodes scapularis*, commonly known as deer ticks. Because the ticks are so small, many people don't notice getting bitten by them. It is estimated that at least half of Lyme disease transmissions come from ticks that are in the nymph stage, when ticks are approximately the same size as a poppy seed.

It's a wonder of nature that something nearly microscopic can pack such a punch to human health. Looked at dispassionately, it's truly fascinating.

If a tick does implant on you, by the time it is an observable size on your body meaning it has engorged itself multiple times its original size by sucking *your* blood chances are it has been on you for around 24–48 hours, long enough to transfer its nasty disease to you. When fully engorged, they just fall off. Even fully engorged with your blood at their full size, ticks are only about the size of a sesame seed.

Theoretically, this entire process can occur without your knowledge. Besides being tiny, ticks hide. These nasty, minuscule parasites seek and implant in warm, dark areas on the body. For example, back of the knees, armpits, the head (that's why ticks like animals so much, they're covered with fur), behind earlobes, and, *ahem*, in even more uncomfortable places where removal becomes something you'd trust to only your spouse or an ER doctor.

Adding insult to injury, before and during the bite, ticks release from their saliva (basically they spit on you) protein compounds that prevent itching and pain. They completely anesthetize the feeding area, meaning you'll never feel them bite, attach, or hang out while feeding on you. Yuck!

The next challenge facing quick detection of Lyme disease: *erythema migrans*, or "the bulls-eye rash." Even though widely recognized as the first sign of infection, it is not much help. The rash may or may not appear from 3 to 30 days after the initial bite. The lag time in the rash presentation allows the Lyme to get into your system. Furthermore, statistical reports on the actual expression of the bulls-eye rash range from 20% to at most 50%. So, at best, 50% of possible cases of Lyme disease exist without the very first early indicator. Not great odds of catching it quickly. I never got the rash or noticed the bite.

Of all the people I know with Lyme, which is roughly 30% of my circle of family and friends, only one person had a rash, my sister Lisa. She had an impressively large bulls-eye on her entire back. It was a sight! In the center of her back was a red circle approximately an inch in diameter. From there, the entire thing radiated out in progressively larger rings: all the way to her shoulders, her waist, and down to the small of her lower back.

Prior to the rash, though, she had no idea she had been bitten by a tick. Lisa was quickly treated with intravenous doxycycline and given subsequent doxy to take orally for 2 weeks. She is fine with no lingering symptoms. Adding one more level of intrigue, Lisa's doctor told her the bite could have been anywhere on her body. The center of the bulls-eye does not necessary indicate the bite zone.

Okay, so we have tiny, sneaky ticks that transmit a nasty disease that are super hard to detect, followed by the primary disease indicator that many do not experience, and if they do, the lag time can be up to a month. How can we get out ahead of this mess? There are a couple ways, so stick with me. Then together we'll unwind this the best we can.

At this stage in the process, if you've been unwittingly bitten and have no evidence of a rash, you're probably tooling around with Lyme disease. This is where you can really run into trouble. And this is where a lot of us who have Lyme in a more chronic fashion got stuck. Because Lyme behaves like a great impostor and the symptoms can be slow to present, without any evidence of stage one, the bite, or two, the rash, there's no reason to think you are infected. So many did not (and still do not) know we are infected. Minor health interruptions get explained away until some sort of apex occurrs. Paralysis, loss of random motor functions, tremendous memory loss, Lyme-induced Bell's palsy, a cornucopia of scary symptoms.

This is more or less where my story begins. I'm old enough that I fall into the lower-awareness, explain-away-until-you-no-longer-can camp. And that's why I opened this book with the advice to be paranoid. Because Lyme disease is so enigmatic and the preliminary cause, the sneaky tick, is so evasive, it can go unnecessarily from a disease that is easily treatable to a real, lasting problem.

The best way I can think to split the difference between being blissfully ignorant until you are beaten down by Lyme or living in chronic fear, is to practice vigilance. The most effective, efficient way to proceed is to create an overall body awareness. I like to call it a Body Baseline. It's an easy-to-remember phrase and the implication is simple. Know what is and is not normal to you and your body.

Dispassionately, critically, and honestly assess yourself, your health, your habits, aches, pains...all that is normal to you and your health, both positive and negative. The purpose of knowing your Body Baseline is, if you experience some of the "ordinary" symptoms of Lyme, you're not initially explaining them away. You're paying attention. Maybe if the fatigue persists, for example, you schedule a doctor's appointment and ask to get tested for Lyme. Conversely, every time you're sore you aren't freaking out that you've contracted Lyme. Maybe you've had tennis elbow for years. Because you are paying attention, you have a heightened awareness, and you're keener to changes in your body and to your health.

REALLY know your body. Be aware of pre-existing patterns. Maybe Monday morning fatigue is something that has always been part of your life. Perhaps you work out three times a week but notice you are sore only after a certain class or resistance training day. These things are normal to you, so not necessarily cause for concern. Get and KNOW your Body Baseline. If you need, write it down. Pay consistent attention to your Body Baseline and any deviations that occur.

It can be as simple as, are you more tired than normal this week? Yes. Well okay, don't panic. Do a mental scan, look at your Body Baseline notes if you've written a log. Have you worked longer hours, are your kids not feeling well and creating more demands than normal? Has a generally busier lifestyle this week pushed you to eating on the run? Have you been eating less-than-nutritious food? Extra stress at work? Perhaps not exercising, or maybe you pushed harder than normal at the gym? All these things add up and may cause you to be off your Body Baseline. Maybe none of the aforementioned are true, and you simply are not feeling like yourself. Make a mental note or write it down. Be aware, and if the changes persist with all things being equal, schedule a doctor appointment or go to a local urgent care and get looked at! Certainly, don't allow yourself to become obsessive and myopic, but a healthy dose of awareness can go a long way.

Clearly, not getting Lyme is most ideal, so employ some prevention techniques. If you're outdoors, before going back into the house, do a "tick check." I do one on myself and the dogs after every walk. The ticks are not always visible, so a quick wipe with a damp cloth helps too. Then put that cloth in the clothes dryer on hot heat for at least 20 minutes. Daily thorough vacuuming is a must, especially with pets. When my nieces and nephews are visiting, we do a "tick check" before coming in the house after being outdoors, EVEN if we were just in the yard. If possible, take a quick shower after being outside, and put the clothes you were wearing in the dryer on high for 20 minutes. New evidence shows this should kill ticks that are possibly attached to clothing. I realize that logistically, this is not always possible but when it is, do so. It's like adding another layer of insurance. Common sense logistics can go a long way. The adage holds true: an ounce of prevention is worth a pound of cure.

Unfortunately, before I became sick, I really did not practice anything I've stated above. I kept the house clean and the animals were always on some sort of flea and tick preventative, but I blew off all other growing concerns around Lyme disease. Cases of Lyme disease and public awareness campaigns were really ramping up in early 2000s, but I was dismissive. Honestly, I thought it was overblown. It seemed like an easy story for the local news outlets to churn. I knew of some cases, but I thought they were the exception, not knowing in a few short years they'd almost be the rule.

And truly, in the back of my mind, I thought "no, not me." I'm an 80s kid, we're tough! We were all outside all day. We were never monitored by adults, we rode bikes everywhere without helmets, we climbed and fell out of trees, and played in the woods until dark. None of us ever had any problems. I've never admitted this, but in the back of my mind I kind of thought anyone who got sick from a little bug lurking in the grass was a sissy. No doubt I was operating from a place of hubris, not being as proactive as I should have.

WAKING UP CRIPPLED

So, what happened to me? Simply put, one morning I woke up crippled, unable to walk.

In mid-May 2011, at approximately 4:00 a.m., I was awoken by excruciating pain in my left hip. The pain was extreme, like nothing I've ever felt. It was so bad, it seemed untrue, foreign; initially I didn't think it was real. I thought I was dreaming. I'm a very deep sleeper and vivid dreamer. For a moment I was lost between worlds. I was extremely confused. It didn't take long for me to fully wake. When I did, the pain instinctively drove me to crunch into a fetal position.

My hip felt like there was a crowbar in the joint socket forcing the bones apart, while hot wax was getting poured into and coating the chasm between the bones. The pressure was unbelievable, and the burning internal fire seemed like a cruel joke. It was so sudden and so intense I could scarcely process what was occurring. Because this appeared to be acute and random, I initially thought to get up, get some water, and walk it off. Pinched nerve, crazy muscle spasm, whatever it was, I assumed it was going to pass as acutely as it presented. I psyched myself up to get moving. I remember slowly pressing my hands on the mattress, coming to sitting, supporting my weight with my right hand as I used momentum and force with my left hand to swing my thighs to the side of the bed. I got my feet to the edge of the bed, placed them firmly on the floor, and executed the standard muscles to stand up.

And, nothing. I got scarcely an inch off the bed and fell back down. Tried again, no success, and again. Alright, I can't stand up, my left hip is hurting beyond comprehension, nothing is computing. As I woke more completely, I could feel my skin becoming flush from the sheer pain. I was starting to freak a little. Still incredulous, I thought I'd try one more time. No dice. At this point I felt I had to wake up my husband and ask for his help.

"Honey, I can't stand up, I need help."

"What do you mean, you can't stand up?"

"...I don't know, I can't stand up, my hip really hurts. Please help me up so I can go get some water."

"Ok..."

Was the gist of the sleepy, in the dark spousal conversation.

My husband, Bob, came around to my side of the bed, took my arm, and helped me to rise from the bed. I did not get much higher than a low squat position. Still, I tried to shuffle forward. One step, two steps. Not really steps, it was more like lurching. I did not really travel forward, all my weight pressing unevenly on Bob. Extreme pain, a total lack of strength, and odder still, a seeming inability to walk. None of these things computed. I ran through it mentally again: I'm in extreme pain, I've lost all power, and I can't stand up to walk. The best thing to do was lie back down and go to sleep. The pain was so intense, there didn't seem to be any other options. Bob helped me lie back down, then went downstairs to get me some water and ibuprofen.

I took the pills, drank the water, then crawled back into the fetal position. I recall longing for sleep so desperately. I remember the odd longing for something beyond sleep. I craved a sensation I never experienced before but somehow knew would deliver me from the pain. I wanted to go to a black abyss; I was looking for a sleep so deep I would become part of an unknown void. Luckily, I was able to fall back to sleep. I drifted off into near euphoria, and I vaguely remember saying or thinking, or both, thank you, to whom I did not know. Just thanks for delivery back to rest. Any respite felt like a gift at that moment.

The morning alarm sounded, 7:00 a.m., approximately three hours later. Bob woke up and asked, "Honey, how's you hip?" I stirred a bit and assessed my status, "The same."

It was the same. Not good. This was not good at all, and was really odd. Still, the show must go on. I needed to get to work; my sense was I could not call in sick. First, it would have been very last minute, and second, what would I say, I woke up lame? No doubt the truth, but it sounded so outlandish. Plus, I was still dumbfounded by the whole situation. I couldn't understand what was transpiring, let alone ask a boss to believe me and forgive me for not coming in to work on such short notice.

Eventually we made our way downstairs. Bob was acting as a human crutch. He got me up out of bed and helped me hobble down the hallway and gimped with me down the stairs. I remember thinking it was as if we were participating in a very depressing three-legged race. The two dogs we had at the time, Shadow, our pit bull who has since passed, and Tyler, our Lab who is still with us, were oddly cooperative. They needed their morning walk, but the jovial behavior and sense of urgency they normally displayed was totally subdued. They were calm and seemed to be moving as slowly as me. Bob got the dogs taken care of and swiftly returned from the walk. He ran down to the basement, retrieved an old pair of crutches, set them in the kitchen for me and asked if he could be of any more help before he needed to jet out the door for work.

As far as I could tell, there wasn't a lot more he could help with. The bathroom is small enough that I could maneuver on my own, using the sink, toilet tank, bathtub, and walls as sort of crutches. I slowly and diligently got ready for work. Somehow, I was able to get ready in a reasonable time. Nothing too memorable, I just recall not feeling well, feeling hot from the excruciating hip pain, and deciding that for today, presentable had to be good enough.

The next thing that really sticks in my mind was getting to the car. Damn! Stick shift! That was not good. Forget not good, it was not possible! Luckily, we had a little green Dodge Dakota pick-up we used for house projects and dump runs. I remember maneuvering on the crutches to the truck and hoisting myself in. I got my right leg and butt propped on the seat, a firm grip on the steering wheel, braced myself then pulled hard to get my painful, seemingly paralyzed left hip and leg flung into the cab.

I felt crappy. The pain was thoroughly distracting and so severe. I could not be sure if I was feeling unwell exclusively as a result of a pain reaction, or if I was also sick. In that moment, it didn't really seem to matter. I recall my most immediate concern was getting safely to work. The drive was just under thirty minutes, and taking back roads seemed prudent. I probably shouldn't have been driving, but fortunately, there was never much traffic on the back roads and I could take it slowly. While I was meandering my way up and down the hilly road and methodically navigating the wide turns, I quieted my mind. I wanted to think clearly and openly about what in the world could be happening. Suddenly I got it, as clear as could be, I bet this is Lyme!

I arrived at work, surprisingly close to on time. I plopped at my desk and organized a few items in preparation for the daily morning meeting. Approximately fifteen minutes later, I crutched back to the conference room. Immediately my boss observed my almost complete immobility and the wincing on my face. She inquired, and I recapped the events of the morning. The day was not terribly full, so provided I could complete the items discussed in the morning meeting, I was free to take leave early. So, I did. I left around 2 p.m. and drove directly to the local urgent care.

I remember checking in at the reception desk at the urgent care facility. I was in so much pain, and it was getting harder and harder to get around. I just wanted to get looked at and get some treatment. I was called back to the exam room where

I was met with a cocky, impatient doctor who, after begrudgingly listening to me recount the day's events, suggested I was overselling my condition. Doctor Douchebag continued to tell me that people (me at that instance) who exercise regularly, who don't have a medical degree or some sort of expertise in kinesiology, tend to overdo it, almost always execute poor form, and end up with severe, often irreversible injuries, "like your hip, for example"...

From there he proceeded to elaborate about the fact that he was a tri-athlete and never suffered injures thanks to his handy-dandy medical degree. I was dumbfounded. I had no idea where his disdain was coming from, furthermore, he hadn't even examined me. He got up to leave the room and while walking out he flippantly stated, "I'll write something for the pain and call it in to the local pharmacy."

Did this asshole think I was pill shopping?

He then added, with an over-the-shoulder condescending glance back, "decrease your activity level, or at least stick to basic at-home workout videos. Average people don't really need to push or demand much from themselves when it comes to exercise."

For a moment I thought I was being punked. It was truly surreal. As if the day hadn't already been strange enough.

"Hey, I'm insured, you're not my primary, you have no idea of my medical history, you are here to provide a service. Test my blood, or refund my co-pay, and hand me back my insurance cards." I spouted toward him as he tried to leave the room. It was hard to exude confidence from lying on an exam table (I was getting very low on energy; pain is exhausting), but I mustered up the best fuck-you attitude I could. And it worked!

Standing in the doorway, he turned around fully. His face somehow simultaneously drooped, scowled, and paled. His body language read, "How dare you advocate for your own interests while in my superior doctor presence?" Yet the words that slid resentfully out of his mouth as he slowly pulled the exam room door closed were, "Fine, I'll send in the nurse to pull a vile." He turned back around, pulled the door shut the rest of the way and left.

Well, that was super odd. I didn't know what to think. Honestly, I didn't care. Presumably his bullshit attitude wasn't going to affect the next steps. The phlebotomist was still going to draw my blood, the blood was going to be tested, and the results were going to be reported. I didn't need Doctor Dickwad to care. I just needed the urgent care practice to follow standard protocol. Soon a nurse entered the room, drew some blood, I signed the necessary medical paperwork, and from there I made my way home.

Not a full two hours later my cell phone rang.

"Jennifer?" inquired the voice on the phone.

"Yes," I replied.

"It's Doctor So & So, you need to go to the pharmacy immediately. I've already called in a prescription for you, it should be there waiting. The levels of the *Borrelia burgdorferi*, the bacteria that causes Lyme disease, are some of the highest I've ever seen. Take the doxycycline as soon as you get the medicine. The instructions state to take with food, but if you haven't eaten, don't worry, you can ignore that for now. If you continue to decline over the next 12-24 hours, go directly to the ER and get intravenous antibiotics."

His attitude was grave and his voice firm, a vast difference from the person with whom I interacted just a short while earlier. The blood results turnaround time was shockingly fast. I thought the lab work would take at least 24 hours. I still don't know how he managed to get them so quickly. Maybe he had a change of heart or simply felt badly about the unprofessional level of service he displayed earlier. Whatever. I had too much on my mind at that point to care.

It was a good-news, bad-news situation. My first reaction was to take delight in his contrite tone. My next reaction was to think I was being petty in my delight, but I felt awful and was close to crippled, so hearing his apologetic tone was a small win. The following thought was "Good! I have a diagnosis." I certainly did not anticipate the challenges ahead. At that point, I was still totally oblivious to the severity of the disease and the potential long-term implications.

So that's how this journey started. Violent pain in the wee hours of the morning, followed by a supportive boss, and an arrogant urgent care doctor who, despite the initial dismissive attitude, got me on the necessary medicine as fast as humanly possible.

I'm sure your story of how and when you found out you had Lyme disease is also unique. But that's not necessarily a good thing. When it comes to being sick, unique is not ideal. The nebulous nature of this disease is exactly why it is so hard to pin down, subsequently leaving many with lingering complications.

The first course of treatment is a long-course prescription of antibiotic, usually doxycycline. I don't remember my daily dosage, but I do remember I was on it for 6 weeks. Yikes! No messing around, none of this "I feel better so I'm going to stop taking the medicine," which I always do. This time I did not even consider going off the antibiotic. Because, well, I didn't feel better. Not at all! In fact, I felt worse and worse.

I was not at all prepared for the battles that were coming and that would last for years. There's a tremendous amount of conflicting information around Lyme and chronic Lyme. Perhaps the only fact that is not up for dispute is that all the information is not yet in. The CDC categorizes the perpetual presence of Lyme in the blood as "post-treatment Lyme Disease." Some doctors call it "chronic Lyme" and other doctors call it "totally in your head", clearly the most enlightened on the subject.

Seriously though, for our purposes, the precise label is not crucial. What is crucial is a proper diagnosis. By proper diagnosis, I mean, what tick-borne diseases are in your blood? The language used for more than one tick-borne disease is "co-infection." I don't have any co-infections. I only have Lyme. There are several other tick-borne infections, and more seem to appear each spring and summer.

The goal of this work is to give you a healthy blueprint to follow and to let you know that you can be stronger than the disease. I'll share with you what foods helped me most and I'll provide you with a basic exercise program to keep you moving and strong.

But first, I'll detail the early days of recovery, how I finally gained the power of perspective, and how that perspective gave me the tools to develop a positive mental attitude. Thank you for the opportunity to share my journey. I hope my condensed knowledge can save you time and get you on the track to feeling the best you can while managing Lyme disease.

THE EARLY DAYS

As luck would have it, the pain in the wee hours of the morning, the doctor visit, the whole story with which you are now familiar, occurred on a Friday. I had the whole weekend to rest, and for that I was relieved. Friday evening, my husband got me set up with blankets and pillows on the couch, and I was free to do nothing but rest and take the medicine.

The first thing I really wanted was to be able to walk. I wasn't able to walk without crutches or a person helping me. I certainly could not, for example, carry a glass of water from the kitchen back to the couch. The fact that I needed to grab from object to object, wall to wall, or needed to rely totally on a crutch or person to facilitate walking was demoralizing. Furthermore, getting around was so painful, I would rather not have done it.

Beyond that, not much about that weekend stuck with me. I know I slept a lot, and if I was hungry, Bob made me some food and probably told me to go back to sleep. I took a sick day that coming Monday. By the end of the day on Monday, I'd be approximately 96 hours in to the treatment. I thought with the rest and antibiotics, I'd be generally back to normal by Tuesday.

Nothing could have been further from the truth. In fact, I felt worse with each passing day. My mobility was just as bad, but now I was SO tired, and my head was...strangely fuzzy. I was really distracted, I couldn't remember anything short term. I dropped words in a sentence, then became so distracted by the loss of the word, I had no idea what I was originally talking about. Worse, none of the normal memory jogs were working. Like walking back in to a room (which I couldn't do anyway) to jog the memory. No mental recourse helped. My mind was a totally dark, blank void. It was disconcerting. My husband would try to lighten the mood by asking if the doctor prescribed me "blond pills."

My mind felt so mushy. I felt like I was floating above myself, disconnected from my body. Ironically, the only thing that helped me stay somewhat present was the extraordinary pain in my hips, which had also spread to my knees. That level of pain kept pulling my fuzzy head back to my physical body. It was all quite strange; I thought I was having an allergic reaction to the medicine. But that didn't really stand to reason, as I'd been on the doxycycline for four days by then. This weird confluence of symptoms seemed to present simultaneously and quickly. I kept spiraling by what felt like the minute: more fatigue, more pain, less mobility, higher confusion. I had not prepared to take any more time off work. I was expected in that Tuesday, and somewhere in my poor reasoning, I thought a return to routine would help force wellness.

Although not in any high functioning condition, I intended to get to work Tuesday. Bob helped the previous night, so the morning would be as efficient as possible. Coffee was prepared, clothes laid out, truck pulled very close to the house, and the alarm clock was set a half hour earlier than normal. I made my way to work, albeit slightly late. When I arrived, my boss was kind in letting me know that it was blatantly obvious that I was not well in any capacity, and that I needed to use more sick time. Before I left, we had a cup of coffee together in her office and I lingered past what was a comfortable time frame, but I needed a rest. Simply executing the morning routine of getting to work sapped me of all energy. I had to recharge before I got back on the road to drive home. During the brief morning at the office, I arranged with HR to take off the remainder of the week, with possibly more time if needed. I'd check in that Friday before 4:00 p.m. to see if I needed to extend the time off request. Though it was only Tuesday and I was still optimistic, part of me knew that, although I was not ready to admit it, I'd be reaching out to HR on Friday. I was exhausted, feeble, and I had the sense my emotions were going to start slipping.

I arrived home mid-morning and was glad to be back. I was beyond depleted. My limbs were heavy, like gravity had increased around my proximal zone. I had little to no fight in me. Lying down was all that really made sense, yet I did not want to go back to that couch. The drab jade green monstrosity of an old school pullout sofa bed represented all that was wrong. The blankets were a disheveled mess, the pillows were depressingly uninviting. The whole room had a strange weighty feeling and smelled, either figuratively or literally or both, like sickness and sadness. I stood there staring at my new hovel, quietly admitting to myself that this was as good as it was going to get for now. I flopped on the couch. As dispirited as I felt, the release from the physical pain quickly superseded the emotional discomfort. I fell in to a deep, long sleep.

Over the course of the next several days, I don't have many more clear memories. I know I slept, took pills, slept more. I was probably sleeping around 16 hours a day. I went to bed early and got up late. I'm using the term "got up" generously. I got out of the sofa bed, cleaned up in the bath (no showers yet, too weak), and returned to the couch. Bob had to deal with everything: house chores, dog care, work, cooking, and helping me get around. I recall him seeming a little stressed, always pressed for time no matter what he was doing. I felt somewhat bad seeing him harried, but I didn't care. I was too depleted to generate any actual emotion.

I was just on the couch. In pain, tired, completely fuzzy in the mind, and drained of any real strength. It was a real chore for me to go from totally supine on the couch, for example, to propped up on pillows on the arm rest. I would get winded and the process took what seemed like a half hour, never mind the pain I endured in my joints while pathetically wigging myself to a semi-propped up position. I'm still incredulous when I think back to how immobilized I was.

It was clear things were not right. Initially, I assumed I'd get on the antibiotics, clear up the infection, and get better. Easy. Done. I falsely thought I'd be back to normal within a day or two, max. I can't really attest where I gathered the simplistic idea that I'd be fine in 24–48 hours. I well could have made it up. I'd been blessed with good health all my life, and I think I was just looking at this disease through that young, healthy lens.

Somewhere around two weeks later—time was askew—I was still living on the couch. I hadn't been able to get upstairs in to bed for weeks. I hobbled from the living room to the bathroom and back. I existed in about 500 square feet of living space, and that was almost more than I could handle. Compounding the discomfort of the pain was the fact that I always felt a little greasy, and gross. I was in too much pain to bathe properly. Normally a bath is an order of luxury and relaxation, but in this case, it was a way to get only kind of clean. Was being disheveled contributing to my demoralized state, or was the outer appearance meeting the inner state? I couldn't really unwind the correct answer to that question, and the truth is, it was probably a combination.

All I knew, with any real confidence, was that I was not as bad off as the crazy people on day time television. One after the other, all day, unrelenting talk shows. The show topics were like the refrain of a bad song. Infidelity, questionable paternity, and the eternal weight loss struggle. The day time entertainment was more than enough to make me think, "Maybe I don't have it that bad..."

Slowly, I could feel that my atmosphere of despair was being cracked by agitation. I was getting sick of being sick, unable to walk, and metaphorically chained to the couch. My contrarian nature was urging me to fight back. For too long now I had psychologically accepted this absolute physical trouncing. I could accept the healing process would take longer and that I was obviously naive about Lyme disease. Fine. But I no longer was going to accept anything else without knowing everything I possibly could about Lyme. Clearly, I had time to read up on the topic. I psyched myself up to get to a sitting position, shimmy over to the end table, and grab the laptop. It took some time and a lot of pain, and by the time I was done I was out of breath and winded. So be it for now, that's what constituted a workout. I let my heart rate recover, then I set up a makeshift table of pillows and blankets around me on the couch, opened the computer, and began.

It took a while, mainly because I did not know what I was looking for. Simply Googling "Lyme Disease" will return a plethora of sites ranging from, loosely speaking, "OMG We're ALL Going to DIE the Government Weaponized Lyme on Plum Island," to "Humans Can't Contract Lyme, You're Not Actually Sick" ...and everything in between. It's not hard to weed out the hysteria, arrive at thoughtful information, then ultimately land on readable medical publications. My primary objective was to discover a plausible explanation for why I had gone from bad to worse.

From the studies and publications I read while trying to objectively relate to my ongoing experience, I surmised I was having a Herxheimer reaction, also referred to as a die-off reaction. When the Lyme spirochetes are being killed by the prescribed antibiotic, the spirochetes (spiral bacteria) fragment into pieces, flooding the bloodstream. The immune system answers the accelerated breakdown of bacteria by producing proteins called cytokines to counteract it. This process is normal and good; it is an indication that the body is doing its job, and it is sometimes accompanied by a symptom spike.

Only a small percentage of people, approximately 15, experience an acute symptom spike (Herxheimer reaction) with the accelerated breakdown of the bacteria and cytokine increase. For those who do, the average reaction time is two to three weeks.

Good, so I was right in line with this. The time frame was correct, and all the add-on sickness I was experiencing were not terribly abnormal. Yes, I was getting sicker, no I was not losing my mind, and it was all a means to an end.

Finding this was a true relief. By all indications, I had another week to go, then I should see an alleviation of the add-on symptoms. From there, if I had no discernable improvement, I planned to go back to the doctor, but I could easily ride out the next week knowing I was on the right healing path.

First victory! I felt less alone, less scared, and my anxiety level relaxed a touch. Provided I basically followed the time frame laid out in the literature I read, I was emotionally satisfied. I had more time to log in this apex of feeling like total crap, but I could manage, knowing there was hopefully relief in sight.

I returned to work three Mondays later. By that point, I had missed 18 business days and used all my sick time, and then some. I was still in rough shape. Thankfully, all the neurological symptoms had subsided. No more confusion, forgetfulness, headache, or extreme fatigue. There had been a crescendo of the illness during the Herxheimer reaction that alleviated with time and rest, then a funnel right back to the original problem: excruciating joint pain that rendered me nearly lame.

I was off the crutches, but barely ambulatory on my own. I could scarcely stand upright. The pain was still strong, and I instinctively hunched to favor the more painful left side. My gait was way off. The disease had attacked the left side most aggressively, so I had a very pronounced limp. Had I not been so sick and almost completely immobilized for the previous three plus weeks, I might have been embarrassed by my new physical presentation.

That's initially what I told myself: I'm not embarrassed, I'm not self-conscious. At my office, the staff was small and family like. Everyone knew what was going on, and it was largely a non-issue. Everywhere else though, I felt like all eyes were on me. And in large part, they were.

I was buckled forward, walking slowly, SLOWLY, left foot dragging. Sometimes to get the left leg completely forward to execute a full step, I had to apply pressure on the back of my left thigh. People couldn't help to look, not look.

Part of my duties at work was end-of-day Post Office drop-off. On the short walk across the street, some offered help to cross, others offered an awkward smile, but most simply evaded eye contact. I did not relish feeling exposed, but I un-doubtedly understood people's discomfort at the sight of me. I know I looked off-putting; my limp was so pronounced and pace so slow, hunch so deep, one may have assumed I was fak-ing. Many in the office complex area didn't know one another by name, but certainly by face. Just short of a month ago, I was seemingly "normal." No limp, no dramatic hunch. People were afraid to ask, and I can't blame them.

Truth is, I was embarrassed and self-conscious. I felt terri-ble holding up the pace of life with my absurdly slow walk and bizarre gait. How long this would persist I didn't know; some are permanently crippled, so I could not rule that out. I felt the spotlight. People were staring, not to be cruel, but it was just weird, I can admit that.

I thought, incorrectly, if I were going to prevent myself from being annoyed by the people around me, I had to put myself in their place. I had to not just intellectually understand their discomfort; I had to feel their discomfort. When I looked more closely in people's eyes, I saw it. It wasn't discomfort, it was pity. That stung. As sick as I had been, and as handicapped as I had become, I hadn't considered that I was deserving of pity.

If at first blush people were feeling sorry for me, then how was I supposed to feel? Forget embarrassed, I should be pissed and resentful. It had been a solid month and I was a poor excuse for ambulatory.

Instantly, the negativity flowed. The "why me" flood gates flung wide open. The sinister comfort offered by such thinking was easy to bathe in. Instinctively, I knew it wasn't a path to anything good, but I didn't care. Wallowing in powerlessness is oddly empowering and totally tempting. Emotions beat out logic, and I hopped on the self-indulgent train and proceeded to feel totally sorry for myself. I wanted my pound of flesh. From whom, I did not know. There was no one to blame, so I just directed my anger at the world, deciding it was well within my rights to be generally unpleasant to everyone.

Thankfully, about a week after the negative spiral began, I had dinner plans with my parents. My mother reminded me that the more time spent in the vicious state of feeling sorry for yourself, the harder it is to untangle. The darker and deeper the rabbit holes you go down, the more you lose perspective and buy your own bullshit. She sternly but lovingly told me to "Have a pity party but keep it short." So I did, and I did.

It took work to pull out of the negativity nosedive, but what's the alternative? Let negativity get the better of me? I couldn't control everything, that was abundantly obvious. There was a nasty disease trying like hell to survive in and take over my body. And at this point it was kicking my ass. There was no denying that. I had a host of new physical limitations, some of which may well be permanent. I had to come to terms with this possibility before I could fully embark on fighting the mental battles.

Truthfully, I had no idea what was in store. I decided to at least stop assuming the worst. For that matter, stop assuming anything. Deal with the known. When I was able to get myself to that bit of psychological stability, I started to reinstate a better perspective. The most obvious truth I grabbed was the fact that I was not terminal. My life was not in jeopardy as a result of this disease. The perils out there are real; there are so many far worse off than me.

I kept looping that one thought through my mind, like a mantra, until the gravity of that truth sank in. In the past I dutifully claimed to practice gratitude, but I don't think I ever actually meant it. I gave myself credit for tossing around profound-sounding phrases without ever actually doing the work. I shudder to think how vapidly I behaved at times before this experience.

A practical way I learned to institute and maintain perspective was to simply take stock. I asked myself, "What do I have, what don't I have?" I asked and answered in the most literal sense and started making a list. Not at all surprisingly, I had WAY more than I did not have.

I have Lyme disease, and I can't walk.

I have access to resources, information, medical care, shelter, clean running water, transportation to medical facilities, I've never been hungry, I have a caring family. The cascade of the haves so overwhelmed the have nots, I was awestruck. I was stunned, and in quiet honesty, I was ashamed I had not ever actually realized how off-balance to the good my life was and is.

I so clearly remember the feeling of pure gratitude. It is easy and probably alright to temporarily be small-minded and selfish. We all have our moments. But since that minor epiphany I make my best, consistent efforts not to hang in an ungrateful mental space. I was sick enough and hobbled enough, THANKFULLY temporarily, that when shown a possible alternative to my blessed life, the power of gratitude rooted deeply in my psyche.

The certitude that I have the tools to unlock and maintain mental strength flooded my mind as powerfully as the disease infested my body. If the price to pay for such a valuable lesson was getting Lyme disease, I was oddly thankful for having gotten sick. Armed with a different attitude, I began to look at my situation in a new light.

I started to ask: What can I do beyond the recommendations of my primary care doctor? What is known, and not known about Lyme disease? There must be more to the story. Truth is, my doctor didn't even warn me about the Herxheimer reaction. This oversight alone made me ponder that perhaps there is more here than meets the eye. By and large I've been blessed with good health, and what ailments I have had until this point were all easily managed with basic care. Until now, I've had no need for questioning a doctor's recommendations or wondering about the limitations of their pre-scribed remedies.

After the onset of my new perspective, I began to more carefully observe myself. I was better able to recognize new, out-of-character habits I was forming. Why, for example, since I'd been diagnosed and, put on antibiotics, had I suddenly be-come a sugar fiend? The strangest new habit: craving soda specifically, Wild Cherry Pepsi!? As a child, I was never al-lowed to drink soda except at a birthday party or at McDon-alds. Soda was a treat, certainly not a beverage option; one drank water or milk, and later in life, wine.

Raised with these habits, it never occurred to me to keep soda in the house. But suddenly and mindlessly, Wild Cherry Pepsi was a new staple that I drank right from the two-liter bottle, no glass required. I was like a zombie for sugar. I remem-ber once being in the kitchen after having eaten a *way*-too-big piece of ooey-gooey chocolate cake, standing half-cocked, lean-ing on the open refrigerator door for support gulping my Cherry Pepsi directly from the liter and abruptly thinking, "How did I get here?" The thought was literal and figurative. Literally, how did I let myself become such a sugar devotee, and figuratively, how did I eat all that cake and jump to greedily drinking the soda before I truly realized what I was doing?

My odd sense was my actions were 50/50: half me, half the pushy disease trying to take over my body. It was a peculiar feeling, but at that moment, I was certain I was correct in my assessment. It felt as if I was eating for it, not me. It was a creepy intuition, and I had no intention of allowing this sym-biotic relationship to go any further. It was time for me to take control.

RECOVERY

The antibiotics are the first responders. First responders come in, kick ass, save your butt, then send you to the hospital. From there on out, you're not their problem, but you're alive, they did their job. Without the first responders, there's no need for secondary or tertiary care. Think of the antibiotic like this: the medicine and doctors stopped the rampant damaging infestation from wreaking more havoc and halted more potential damage. Was it enough? Will there be little leave-behind gifts from the Lyme bastards? Maybe, maybe not.

I finally finished the antibiotic course in early July. I was able to stand with crooked posture on both feet without assistance, and I was able to plod along. Neither was great, but it was a measurable improvement. I was back to regularly walking the dogs, albeit slowly, but that was the extent of my activity and ability. I wanted to get back to exercising.

My previous weekly routine was a mixture of a couple five-mile runs and one or two group fitness classes after work. I kept thinking, "Okay, next week", I was still relatively happy to have made such drastic improvements and I wasn't yet thinking, "Something here is not right." Still, July came and went with no noticeable improvement. I hit a plateau. My joints complained some, but in general, I was feeling good. But that left hip, though, boy that guy was a problem. It was as if from the waist down I had gone from a healthy 37-year-old woman to a just-barely-ambulatory octogenarian.

I was getting impatient. I decided I was going to tough out the joint pain and weaknesses. Surely some of this was mental. From how sick I had been to now was a drastic improvement. I thought maybe some of the slow-down in progress was me babying myself, being overly cautious, fearful, nervous. I decided it was time to start pushing the envelope. I convinced myself the only way to get back on top of being fit and strong was to work through the last of the hip limitations.

There are plenty of senior citizen runners. Last fall, one of my good friends finished the NYC marathon at 82. I'll just take it slow, like them, and eventually, voila; I'll get moving, and everything will be back to normal.

One evening, I put on my favorite running capris, laced up the running shoes that had been sitting dormant in the closet for almost five months now—no dog (I was smart enough to know that was a bad idea!)—cued up a playlist on the MP3 player, and out the door I went.

With my ugly left-favoring posture and strange gait, I started up the street. One foot diligently in front of the other. I couldn't even move fast enough to get my heart rate up. But on I shuffled. The fantasy was that with each stride, my hip joints would loosen up, power would grow inside, the "Chariots of Fire" theme song would magically emanate from and around me, and I would be buoyed to mental and physical victory. I liked that story. I visualized that story. But it didn't happen.

The truth was my physical limitations and pain were clearly in charge, and I barely scraped forward for less than a tenth of a mile. I had to stop. I was overcome with pain and a strange void of strength in my hips. I would have sat on the ground, but being able to get back up was not something I would have bet money on.

So, I just stood there, on the side of the street. Hunching even more now toward the really bad left hip, wincing. I wondered how weird it would be to hitchhike home.

Summer was waning early that year. It was still warm, but I noticed the smell of fall in the air. I tried to fake a pensive look, pretending to be pondering what changes the new season may bring. I was trying to feel and appear less odd, randomly standing around. There I stood, with an expression that was a mixture of real pain and fake intellectual curiosity. I couldn't but help roll my eyes at myself and wonder exactly how ridiculous I appeared in that given moment. "Good god, I'm an idiot and that was a terrible idea!"

But standing I was, so good enough for now; time to walk home very slowly and very carefully! It took about 45 minutes to traverse the tenth mile, but I got there. Alright, so then I knew what not to do.

I paid for that poor excuse of a run for about three weeks. I set myself back to being almost unable to walk. I was even off the morning dog walk until the end of the month. The mindset of "next week, next week, I'll be set to return to my normal, previous life," was fading. It became clear to me I had to reassess everything I knew about my physical being. Although I knew I might have to consider a new physical paradigm for myself, I was not ready to accept it. That foolish run brought me a little closer to acceptance. I could not remain sedentary, but I could not exercise in any way I was familiar with. What were my options? I was at a loss, but one thing I was sure of; I needed to get my hips rechecked by my doctor.

Shortly after the unsuccessful run, I made an appointment with my primary care doctor. During the visit, he was starting to betray a little worry around the hip recovery. He referred me to an orthopedic specialist who wanted a closed MRI to get a look at my hips. The slow recovery of the hip joints, especially the left, was becoming cause for concern. Man, that F'ing hip hurt, like always, and badly.

The process of doctor visits quickly became a grind. The structure of insurance companies' referral system of prerequisites becomes time-consuming. Although the doctors know exactly what sort of tests they need to perform to look for answers, it was necessary to go through each step determined by the insurance company to ensure reimbursement. Miss a step, run the risk of self-pay.

To comply, sometimes I had to travel to NYC or Albany to see a specialist. Long tiring days, more missed work, painful exams, long needles injecting contrast dye in the joints. Blah, blah, blah...and suddenly between doctor's visits, work, and trying to maintain basic ambulatory status, fall had arrived, and cold weather was on the way.

The primary problem the orthopedic specialist was looking for was a torn labrum in the left hip joint. Their theory, both the primary and orthopedic doctor, was the severity of the inflammation had caused a breakdown in the cushioning where the head of the femur inserts into the pelvis.

The final consultation with the orthopedic doctor was on a cold, wet day. It was a rainy, grey, dark-by-5:00 p.m., winter-around-the-corner kind of a day in upstate New York. The weather sticks out in my mind because I became sorer, I had discovered, in the damp cold, and I was getting nervous about the impending winter.

Besides increased discomfort and reduced range of motion that seemed to follow the nastier weather, I developed a fear of falling. It's slippery here in the winter, and I really didn't think I could absorb the shock of a fall. I could feel an anxiety creep that was making me uncomfortable. I did not want new neurosis sneaking in to my psychological profile because of this disease. I had enough new problems to solve. I took a moment before I opened the car door.

Breathing deeply, I did my best to calm the tirade of unrealized what-ifs that, if left unattended, could prove to make me bonkers. I resolved to just take it slow, now and as the winter months approached. I would exercise caution, move deliberately, and things should be alright. I calmed myself down with one last deep breath, slowly opened the door, judiciously placed my feet on the ground, and made my way into the large facility.

Doctor Schneider laid out the summary of findings: luckily no tears, which meant no surgery, but oodles of inflammation that was causing the head of the femur to rub and irritate at the pelvis insertion. The damage was way more pronounced on the left than the right, but both were considered arthritic joints. Over time, deterioration was to be expected. In the meantime, if something hurts, don't do it.

That was it. That was it? No recommendations, no words of wisdom? Will it go away, what about the Lyme, is this permanent damage, how, when will I return to normal? In a nutshell, he told me that inflammation is inflammation; the cause of the damage as it related to his specialty was a secondary concern. His medical mandate: "Do I need to operate or not?" In my case, the answer was no, so his only advice was, "Don't irritate it further."

Ugh! All that time for "If this hurts, don't do it"? I had higher hopes of better answers! Desperate babble left my lips before I really gave myself permission to talk. I started giving him a summary of what I was capable of only six months ago, where I was currently, driving at the idea I wanted to be back to where I was and more.

He half listened. His face had a bored look, though his body language was kind and mildly sympathetic. I clearly was not the first patient to express the "but, but, but..." sentiment to him.

Dr. Schneider took a deep breath, exhaled as he leaned closer, and looked me square in the eyes and said, "Look, by your physical condition I can see you are someone who has been athletically active most of your life. I can confidently tell you, you will not be able to return to most, if any, of those activities, not without pain, not in any productive manner, and not without serious consequences. I can't give you much advice on what to do; that is not my scope of practice. I will advise: do not hurt the joints any more. I'm sorry to be the one to tell you this, but your options are now limited."

With that he stood, my file still open in his broad hands. His posture was impressively erect, shoulders back. He was a wide, tall man. He looked down at me with a half-smile and closed my file. It was clear the appointment and the discussion were over.

I felt sad on the way out of his office. My head was hung low in dejection. So low that my most vivid memory of that entire office complex was the brown tweed color of the Berber carpet. What kind of sadist has medium-pile Berber carpet in an office where most of the patients are in a wheel chair or on crutches? I wanted to hate him, his stupid face, his perfect posture, and his damned Berber carpet.

But it wasn't his fault. He was just the last stop. All standard medical options needed to be explored in the aim of getting better. Thanks to the doctor's honesty, I had to square with myself the fact that things had changed, permanently. The truth is, it could have been worse.

From all the doctors I had seen, I noticed a refrain. It went something like this: we don't know a ton about left-over damage from Lyme Disease, furthermore some (in 2011 it was most) medical professionals don't believe Post Treatment Lyme exists. Even though more than half of the proteins associated with Lyme are showing as reactive and the Lyme bands are still present in your blood, we consider you not infected, at least not to the level where more antibiotics would be prescribed, so we have no further treatment advice. We can see evidence of arthritis in the hips, do not participate in any activities that would exasperate an arthritic condition, that's the best we can do. I was not offered a panacea, but I had good care, I trusted what information the doctors could offer, and knew what not to do.

By December 2011, seven months in to this debacle, I had come to the end of the road. Since May, I had come quite far, but I didn't want to accept I was going to be just kind of alright. Being able to walk was a treat. I'm not saying that casually. I mean it, and I was grateful, but I was still young. And up until seven months earlier, I was pretty athletically active. I was having a hard time folding my cards and deciding this was good enough. I decided my mandate was to explore if I could bolster my body with good food and exercise kowing that everything about exercise with which I was previously familiar was out the window.

STARVE IT, NOURISH YOU

I dove in to the concept of playing with my diet before embarking on the exercise journey for practical reasons, the most obvious being that my hips were still quite fragile. I was ambulatory and free of the crutches, but if I walked too long, I'd pay with pain. If I tried to walk at a brisk pace, I'd buckle over to the left. I never fell all the way down, but I came close a couple times. My joints were simply so weak they could only take so much force before giving out. I used to feel like those vintage toys that stood on a small pedestal. Some of you more seasoned readers may remember them. I recall a horse on a small wooden pedestal where you could press the bottom or squeeze the sides and the horse would go limp, and just hang, sort of suspended. My hips behaved similarly to that old toy. My hips, predominantly the left would kind of slip, give way, I'd jerk a bit, usually to the left and sort of back. I learned the best way to manage this was to stop walking, find my balance, reset, and carry on. Naturally, I was nervous about adding in physical activity. So, food first.

I started thinking about the strong drive to sugar I had in the early recovery stages, which still lingered, albeit not as intensely. The first thing I did was to keep a food journal for a week. A food journal is crucial to ensure accuracy. It's easy to forget or overlook something we just pop in our mouths. Writing down everything honestly and thoroughly can be eye opening. Beverages and what goes in those beverages must be included. For example, sugar in coffee, soda with whiskey, honey in tea. It all matters. It is prudent to know exactly everything you are consuming, and knowing will make change, if needed, an easier task.

My first discovery was that I was consuming a lot more sugar than I realized. I don't think I initially noticed my overall increased sugar consumption because my intake spiked so dramatically in the beginning that when I decreased consumption, it was already from an abnormally high metric. My calibration was off.

What was going on here? Sugar obviously is delicious, and really pleasing to eat, but I had a suspicion that there was more behind sugar being my new favorite food group.

Simply put, the *borrelia burgdorferi*, the spiral-shaped Lyme bacteria, thrive on glucose. You are the host to the parasite, and it wants sugar. DO NOT FEED IT! Drastically reducing sugar intake will help starve the spirochetes, and that's what we want.

Tamping down sugar intake is not a magic cure, and you will not feel instantly better. But rather, you will strengthen your body and weaken the disease. Every positive tool you give yourself is a win.

In addition to removing an easy fuel source for the spiro-chetes to access, reducing sugar will have overall health benefits. Sugar reduction has been linked, almost undisputedly, to inflammation reduction. So, it stands to reason if you have Lyme Disease that is attacking and flaring up your joints, don't help the damned disease. Give yourself a fighting chance.

It is not my aim in this book to delve into the topic of sugar, especially because I think we all know that the health hazards of consuming too much sugar are far and wide. What I will say, however, is that reducing overall sugar intake will have a spectrum of health benefits in addition to helping you beat back Lyme.

I think the fundamental problem in the modern diet with sugar is that most of us are unaware of just how much we're actually consuming. Sugar is hidden everywhere. Considered a nonessential nutrient, sugar doesn't have an RDA (recommended daily allowance), but rather a recommendation for a maximum daily allowance (MDA). According to the American Heart Association, the MDA (maximum daily allowance) for women is 25 grams (6 teaspoons), and men 36 grams (9 teaspoons). Actual average consumption is 178 grams, or 42 teaspoons a day. Seems like a lot of sugar. Surely, you're thinking, not me!

But sugar hides everywhere. For example, a 12 ounce can of cola has 39 grams (10 teaspoons) of sugar. Have a glass (8 oz.) of orange juice and you'll add another 18 grams (5 teaspoons) of sugar. Add the afternoon pick me up a coffee-cappuccino treat and you're in for at least another 110 grams (27 teaspoons). These 3 drinks are around 167 grams (42 teaspoons) of sugar, and this example is nothing extraordinary, and we didn't even touch food yet. If you think you're exempt from that 42 tea-spoon a day average, think again. Sugar is just ubiquitous in daily life and a lot of the excess consumption is unintentional. So let's just take a step back and make a few changes.

Total elimination of sugar is a daunting task, and I'm not advocating for complete removal of sugar. Significant reduction, however, is not insurmountable, is extremely beneficial, and can be accomplished simply by paying a little more attention. Below are five easy steps that will help you make great strides in reducing sugar intake.

Reduce Sugar in 5 Easy Steps:

1) Eliminate alcohol and sweets. For many, me included, fine wine, delicious baked goods, or a rich ice cream sundae makes life worth living. The thought of total and indefinite abstinence from booze and sweets may make you gasp and is not realistically sustainable. If you love a dessert, a sweet treat, wine, beer, or mixed drink, FINE! Allow it, but sparingly once a week, for example. I believe we all know, deep down, we've gotten WAY too liberal with the amount of sweets we allow ourselves to eat. At the office, the mid-morning meeting is accompanied by a coffee and a pastry. The 3 o'clock crash rears its head and we take "just a little bite" of that whatever is in the break room while fixing the afternoon coffee. We make a little excuse, as if justifying the consumption will negate the biological effects. It does not, and we all know it. Downshift the consumption to a once a week treat. Your body will thank you.

2) Eliminate soda and sports drinks. No exceptions. Do not replace soda with diet soda! Drink water! Water, water, and more water. Seltzer is acceptable too, just be careful not to fall for slick labels. Do not buy anything other than plain seltzer, squeeze a little lime or lemon in the drink if you'd like. It seems like beverage companies are noticing slight changes in consumer behavior and are trying to keep up. Of late I've noticed a lot of beverages on the shelf that are promoted as healthy. First tip: if it says anything on the label like "zero calories" or "zero sugar" or "sparkling..." beware, something is UP! There is no doubt some version of an "*ose*" in there—dextr*ose*, fruct*ose*, sucr*ose* —ose is the suffix used to denote a sugar. Don't bother, your body doesn't need it, don't pay for gimmicks. Water and plain seltzer are the best.

3) Eliminate all fancy coffee. Replace with regular coffee with a little milk, if you like, but no added sugar. Might not taste as good, but so what! Coffee is a stimulant and should be used as such. Forget all the hoopla around coffee. Drink it when you need to and forget the rest. This might give your wallet a little break, too.

4) Eliminate fruit juice. It's scarcely juice and mostly sugar. Look at the nutrition labels, you might be surprised at how little nutrition is in the "juice." I'm going to provide a recipe for an improved way to get your vitamins from fruit while still getting the benefits of the natural fibers.

5) Eliminate processed food. Skip the frozen food and convenience isles. All this food is packed with sugar and so-

dium and is light on nutrition. Get into the habit of reading nutrition labels AND ingredients on the products you buy in the grocery store. Don't rely on the flashy information on the front of the package—*"ONLY 75 CALORIES PER SERVING"* sort of stuff. Ignore all that, it intentionally highlights the "good" news and leaves out most of the actual information. You may be shocked at the amount of sugar you are unintentionally consuming. Don't forget, the ingredients are listed in order of most to least. Your first trip or two to the store will take a little longer than normal, but it will be second nature before you realize it.

By simply executing the above five steps, you will make great strides in bringing you diet to a better balance. Now that we've taken away the spirochetes' preferred food source, let's give back to your body to keep it at the optimal level for fighting.

I am not an evangelist for any diet over another. Gluten free, paleo, vegetarian, vegan, ketogenic, Atkins all have a place and a purpose. Moreover, if your doctor has instructed you to ascribe to or, conversely, to avoid a certain way of eating, listen to your doctor. I am simple in my approach to eating. Purchase and cook nutritious food, virtually nothing processed, focus on protein, vegetables, and complex carbohydrates.

Equally important to what we eat is how we eat. Modern society tends to be in a hurry. People wear busyness as a badge of honor and stopping to eat has, for many, risen to the level of a transgression. It's loony, but understandable, that we won't even allow a small respite in our day to eat. Study after study demonstrates that eating on the run is counterproductive. Almost without exception, those who regularly eat on the run underestimate the amount of food eaten while simultaneously overestimating the quality of food eaten.

Furthermore, eating on the run decreases satiety, meaning you enjoy the food less-if at all-which allows one to easily forget that they ever ate. This, in turn, leads to more snacking. Worse yet, the subsequent snacking is typically on junk food, not on foods like carrot sticks or nuts. The theory is that the decreased satiety sets up a deprivation feedback loop in the mind. The result is, an "I deserve this treat" mindset even though most of what has been eaten over the course of a day, week, or longer is closer to "treat-like" food rather than nutritious food.

Given the incessant tasks allotted to the modern employee, let alone the added responsibilities of family and household, it's no wonder this is happening. It needs to stop though. With a little kindness to yourself, and minor planning once a week, we can get about 80% better. That 80% better means that five days a week, we take a little time out of the day to stop and eat.

To break the bad habits of eating on the run and mindless eating, I put myself on a food schedule. It has been tremendously helpful in making me more conscientious in relation to food and it's not nearly as stringent as it sounds. Being organized around food has allowed me to make better dietary choices. The improved nutrition underpins a foundation of feeding my body good stuff to help it stay strong while Lyme tries to make me weak.

My schedule is hectic, so I know how challenging it can be to stay on track. My strong suit is that once I implement a system, I'm pretty good about sticking with it. My weakness is first getting the system in place. It took some trial and error, but in time, I got this system down to a science. And don't forget the 80/20 rule.

If for the week you're 80% on target, that's five, maybe six days where you'll comply, leaving one day to be a little lackadaisical. I say lackadaisical rather than "cheat," because here we're discussing diet in relation to management of a chronic disease. If your willpower slips, it's a little different than if we were discussing diet exclusively for weight loss. I mention the 80/20 rule because perfection can be the enemy of progress. If you start off with the intention of absolute perfect adherence, you may not stick with a healthier eating plan for the long term. Think marathon, not sprint.

The Eating Schedule:

6am Wake Up
(Wake up same time within 30 minutes each day)

Dilute 4 ounces of blend (recipe below) with 4 ounces of water, drink.

1-2 cups coffee, black or with milk

Get ready for work/the day

11am Mid-morning snack

Choose ONE from:

- Unsalted (you'll get used to it) Nut mix: cashews, almonds, Brazil nuts; serving size 1/2 cup

- Plain yogurt; serving size 1 cup

- Carrot sticks cut from whole carrot (baby carrots are just creepy); 4-5 sticks

- 2 hardboiled eggs

- **Drink water**

1-2pm Lunch (This doesn't mean you take an hour to eat. It's a time frame—to eat you only need 15-30 minutes—just make sure to STOP what you are doing, then eat. If you're driving, pull over for 15 minutes; if you're at your desk, STOP "multi-tasking" for 15 minutes).

Meal 1: 3-4-ounce chicken breast (seasoned to your liking, but not BBQ sauce because it's a source of a lot of hidden sugar; I have a list of condiments to avoid in the next section) on WHOLE GRAIN bread (eat only complex carbohydrates, and eat them sparingly, list on these too). Again, READ nutrition labels and ingredients. Many products have a healthy veneer but are not. INCLUDING PRODUCTS FROM HEALTH FOOD STORES. Be vigilant—no exceptions. The best whole grain bread I found is "Heidelberg Baking Company Multi-Grain." It is delicious and full of good ingredients, all of which you can read and pronounce! Add avocado slices, tomato, and alfalfa sprouts. Really pile on the sprouts; they're tasty, low in calories, and full of vital vitamins and minerals your body needs to remain strong.

Meal 2: The big salad: greens of beets, kale, and dark lettuce (romaine or green leaf), chopped pepper, onion, tomato, avocado, 2-3 sliced hard-boiled eggs. Olive oil and red wine or apple cider vinegar (not balsamic, too much sugar) to taste. I like to add garlic powder, too.

Meal 3: Out to lunch? Order 2-3 eggs, sauerkraut, kimchi, coleslaw, or cottage cheese in lieu of the home fries. No toast. Add a side salad with olive oil & red or apple cider vinegar.

Meal 4: 3-4 ounces chicken breasts (seasoned to your liking, again, no BBQ sauce), 1/2 sweet potato, and serving from the salad above

Drink water and or a cup of coffee.

Mid-day snack 3-4 pm (only if you're hungry, or if you're craving something on the no-no list)

Revisit the mid-morning snack list, then swap out: if you had an egg, have nuts now. Also, if you're having an afternoon craving or crash, have the nuts. Nuts are delicious and full of good fats, which will help to tamp down a sugar craving and make you feel satisfied. If you had the yogurt, then now have the carrots. Use common sense and good judgement. Initially, write down what you're eating to help you keep track.

7-8pm Dinner (Again, remember to stop what you are doing and only eat)

3-4 ounces of a protein source (fish, poultry, eggs, red meat, pork, or organ meat) cooked to your liking.

Add: 2-3 servings of vegetables, either fresh or frozen fresh. I always keep frozen veggies on hand; they're good to have, BUT DO NOT buy any that are pre-seasoned. Plain, plain, plain is what you want. You're a good cook, do the flavoring yourself. Know and control what you're eating.

Add: Serving of rice and beans. This is a magically nutritious combination, and the seasoning possibilities are endless. OR Half or whole sweet potato, depending on size; some get big!

This is a well-balanced diet focusing on simple food. Although it may seem dull, it is far from it. There's great variety and endless flavoring possibilities. Purchase plain, plain, plain, then you season to your liking. You're controlling your intake of sugar, salt, and chemicals. See my list of 10 condiments to avoid. Some of the most commonly used condiments are PACKED with sugar, salt, and often preserving agents you can do without.

Here's that breakfast blend:

8 ounces dark berries

1 medium orange

¼ cup pineapple or ½ grapefruit

Roughly chopped ginger, not peeled, to taste. Chop approximately 2 inches. Start with less, especially if you're not accustomed to ginger, as it's potent and I don't want you to hate your first batch.

In a standard 48-oz blender, the fruit above should fill the jar about half way, add only water to the mix, stop at 36 ounces to avoid a volcano of juice exploding on your counter top. Blend, and that's it! You have your breakfast blend for the week. Tons of must-have vitamins for bone and joint health and lots of natural fiber, ginger for digestion, and a low impact on the glycemic index.

Pour four ounces in a glass every morning, then fill the glass to the top with water for a little more dilution. Drink! This should fill you up, along with a cup of coffee or two, for at least 4-5 hours. If initially you're noticing you're hungry before time for the mid-morning snack, add a tablespoon of plain yogurt to the morning juice blend.

Once you have been on this diet for a week or two, your hunger levels should be relatively steady. The caloric consumption is plenty (about 2,000), it is well timed, and full of nutrient-dense food that your body is putting to good use. Furthermore, the stepped-down sugar consumption should allow for more stable insulin levels. Insulin spikes send signals to the brain to release the hormone that causes the hungry feeling. Hormones are largely responsible for the "I'm starving" feeling that in turn often leads to grabbing at any available food. A lot of, but not all, hunger signals are driven hormonally and are not coming from a truly empty belly.

With better insulin signaling, you will be better able to exercise control of food choices. Generally, you should not have that desperately hungry feeling. Rather you most likely should simply feel like you're getting a little hungry. Most often you will have the sense that your body has taken what you fed it, put it to use, has digested the fuel, and it will soon be time to give it more fuel a la food.

If you are more hungry than normal, remember that it's OK to be a little hungry. You are not going to starve. We are blessed to live in a time of such abundance that it seems like our barometer of what it means to be truly hungry is a bit askew. According to a 2017 report by the United Nations Food and Agriculture Organization, the average American consumes between 3,000-3,600 calories per day. At the top end, that is 1,600 calories over the generally accepted 2,000-calorie threshold, which is potentially high considering the average person's overall activity level.

For perspective, 1,600 calories is 3 Big Macs. This is a lot of unneeded caloric consumption; perhaps being a little hungry isn't the worst thing, and it may be necessary for a proper reset of the digestive system.

Remember, there are people all over the world and in our backyards who live every day with bona fide food scarcity. Keep them in mind next time you proclaim, like we all have, "I'm starving." You're not starving, I have never gone unwillingly hungry, chances are you haven't either, and it would do a lot of us a bit of good to reserve the use of the term starving for its actual denotation.

I say this not to be harsh, but rather because I want to see all my readers help themselves feel better. Improving one's diet will have tremendous long-term benefits, but initially it can be a rude awakening, and maybe a little shocking to the body. Generally speaking, the American diet isn't really helping us to operate at optimal levels. Instituting some of these changes can be challenging, both mentally and physically. I'd be heartbroken if some of us were unsuccessful as a result of a few hunger pangs. Your body will adjust, and a few hunger pangs are not a big deal, but rather a sign that your body is working, and using the nutritious food it needs, wants, and is now receiving.

A new eating schedule and a different diet, may feel like just one more task to add to your already full time schedule. However, you owe it to yourself to arm your body with the best nutrition to fight Lyme, so you can get and stay feeling better. Below is the system I use to set myself up for the week. It is efficient, painless, and allows for a solid foundation of well-prepared nutritious food for the week without making for yet another project.

From driving to the grocery store to completion, total time should be no more than 2 hours. I need to add that, since I first started writing this book, Bob has completely taken over the household task of grocery shopping, so my load here is cut in half!

Make A Grocery List!!!

1) Grocery shop once a week. Same day, approximately same time.

2) Upon arrival home, prepare food for the week.

A) Preheat oven to 350-375F, place foil on baking sheet (the fewer dirty dishes, the better!), spray lightly to prevent sticking, place sweet potatoes in oven, bake approximately 1 hour.

B) Start water to hard boil eggs.

C) Warm a nonstick pan, melt a little butter or olive oil, place chicken breasts in pan cook on medium heat to prevent burning and allow you to attend to other foods.

D) Rinse vegetables in preparation to rough chop.

E) Water should be boiling now. Safely place eggs in one at a time in water, careful not to splash.

F) Most likely time to flip chicken breasts.

G) Start rough-chopping vegetables. Purchase the best-looking, most seasonal veggies. You don't have to have all the vegetables all the time. Use your judgement; you know what you're doing!

H) Chicken might be almost done; check it, then return to chopping vegetables. For salad and vegetable storage, either combine in a large Tupperware and take smaller portions to work or store all separate and combine as the week goes along. This is up to you.

I) Check sweet potatoes, flip. They are definitely baking if you can smell their sweetness.

That should take no more than an hour and you'll finish with the major foundation for your entire week of eating. If you send the kids to school with lunches, just increase the amount of food. These foods are good for the whole family.

The Must Haves:

Vegetables:

- Alfalfa sprouts

- Beans

- Beets and beet greens

- Broccoli

- Carrots

- Cauliflower

- Kale

- Peas

- Spinach

- Sweet potatoes

Fruit:

- Apples
- Citrus
- Blueberries
- Cherries
- Grapefruit
- Kiwifruit
- Oranges
- Pineapple
- Raspberries

Meat:

- Beef
- Beef liver
- Chicken
- Salmon
- Sardines
- Tuna

Dairy:

- Eggs

- Plain yogurt

- Milk

Nuts & Legumes:

- Almonds

- Brazil nuts

- Peanuts

- Walnuts

Fermented and Fun:

- Ginger

- Kimchi

- Red cabbage

- Sauerkraut

Condiments to avoid:

- Ketchup

- Mayonnaise

- BBQ sauce

- Balsamic Vinegar

- Salad dressing

- Honey mustard

- Cold cuts

- Pre-packaged foods (flavored noodles, rice; buy plain and flavor yourself)

- Spaghetti sauce

- Flavored yogurt (buy plain, don't be fooled by all the new popular brands/flavors)

Complex Carbohydrates:

- Sweet potatoes. Great plain or with a dash of your favorite hot sauce.

Sweet Potato Spread: Mix fresh chopped garlic, 1/2 sweet potato, 2 tablespoon plain yogurt, use as a dip or instead of mayonnaise, ketchup.

- Beans! All Beans! I LOVE beans!!

- PLAIN Oatmeal, steel cut or rolled oats. Instant is acceptable too, but careful to not overcook. For flavor enhancement, add cinnamon and or a teaspoon of local honey.

- Radishes, YUM!! Wash, slice, or eat whole!

- Chickpeas (technically a bean!) YES! Add to a salad or make hummus!

GETTING STRONGER

Next mandate: Move Baby Move!

By late December 2011, I had gotten my diet in better order for about 3 full weeks. I was starting to feel a little more alive, a touch more whole. Looking back, I can now see that although I was grateful to be doing as well as I was comparatively to the beginning, I was quietly harboring a general sadness. I felt like a kid that got picked last or not at all for the team. Physically, I felt like I got left behind. For example, during Christmas parties and various holiday gatherings, I couldn't dance and be generally silly with my friends and family. I was mobile and getting around on my own two feet, but I was otherwise very limited. That year I didn't go to the city for our annual trip (NYC is the best during the holiday season!), because it was just too much getting around for my current level.

All things considered, none of this is the worst fate by any measure, but I wanted more. I missed moving freely, without pain, or perhaps more importantly, without fear of the pain that was always just around the corner. Still, toward the very end of December just before the New Year, I remember feeling a little mightier inside. Maybe it was the improved diet, maybe not. Maybe it was all psychosomatic, maybe it was all biological, maybe it was a combination. Certainly, I did not care. All I knew was, I was more alive each day and I had every intention of building on that.

There was no doubt in my mind I needed to get my body moving. Being largely sedentary for over a half a year now had taken its toll on my body. I was basically fighting atrophy from two fronts. Lyme kicked my ass and left my joints generally sore and my hips nearly unbearable, which in turn promoted a lot of inactivity. The end result was compounding weakness. I asked myself, what's a girl to do?

Only one option: Exercise, Exercise, Exercise! I needed to get moving, and so do you. I know what you're thinking, "What the hell is she talking about, exercise?" "Fat chance, lady!" "You're crazy!" Something like that, right?

But never say die! We have the gift of water! Water will take pressure off your joints, provide buoyancy to allow freer movement than on land, and will create resistance promoting muscular development. It will take time, but it will work!

Visualize your muscles as if they are duct tape around your sore weak joints. With a dutifully executed, smartly planned exercise program, you will realize the power of incremental progress. You will be delighted and shocked at the extent to which a well-developed muscular system will assist in pain alleviation and emotional empowerment.

Hurts to move? Some discomfort is going to be a necessary evil that may never fully alleviate. You are not alone, and worse than exercise-associated discomfort is progressive deterioration from being sedentary. Don't cede all your potential power to the disease. Don't help it beat you. Baby steps every day will bring you further than you could ever imagine.

This is exactly what I did: Find a local gym, YMCA, university, etc. with a pool. JOIN NOW!

1) Stop giving all shits about what you, me, or anyone looks like in a bathing suit. Yes, vanity rears its ugly head all the time.

2) Set a time and day to get in the water that works for your schedule. Time-block that ONE HOUR, twice a week, and stick to it. (Need time to change, dry off, and change again, thus an hour.)

3) Start!

The Workout:

Warm-up: Walk or lightly jog, depending on your cardiovascular fitness, from one end of the pool to the opposite 4 times. The goal should be to get your heart rate up and your blood flowing. Rule of thumb: if you were talking with someone during the warm-up, you should be slightly winded, but still able to talk between breaths. If you can speak freely and are not feeling breathless in any way, you are going too easy on the warm-up laps; if you're winded and gasping for air, you're pushing way too hard. Find the sweet spot and enjoy the water, and work!

Lower Body:

Standing arm's length from the wall of the pool, right hand on the edge, plant your right foot firmly (really feel your toes engaged with the pool bottom), stand tall and firm on that right leg, squeeze your belly button in toward your lower back, spine tall and nice erect posture with chest open, then place your left hand on your waist.

Now, stay erect and tall in the upper body (think actively engaged muscles), from here kick the left leg out to the side. The muscle group you're working here is the outer part of the hip (abductors). Repeat 10 times.

Next, return to the posture, fix any sagging, make sure your belly is still tight, spine tall, NOW kick forward, working the top of the thigh (quadriceps). Repeat 10 times.

Next, check back on your form, still standing tall, right leg still firm, belly zipped in to back. Good! NOW kick back, working the back of the thigh and butt (hamstrings and gluteus maximus). Repeat 10 times.

These three exercises, repeated for ten "repetitions" each, are considered a "set."

Switch sides, same points to highlight. Left hand is secure on side of pool, left leg is firm, toes grip pool bottom. Clear your mind, focus only on your form, then the muscle groups you are isolating to get the most out of the exercise.

Repeat all three ranges of motion for ten repetitions. Side, forward, back.

Then check in with how you feel. Float around a little. Sore? Taxed? That's okay, enjoy the water for a little bit more, call it a win, and look forward to the next workout.

Still have some energy? Great!

Repeat the lower body set, right then left one more time.

The goal is three sets on each side.

Upper Body:

Move to a deeper part of the pool. Ideally, the surface of the water would be just above your shoulders.

Start with the feet awareness. Both are planted firmly on the bottom of the pool, each toe gently spread and pressing into the floor. Legs hip-width apart, slight bend in the knee, arms wide open, palms facing out (fingers together creates more resistance than fingers spread wide. Play with finger placement in relation to your upper body strength). You're a firm, strong but relaxed **T** in the water. From here, bring your palms together in front of the body. Feel the front of the shoulders, chest, and possibly biceps working. Open arms back to **T**. When opening the arms back to **T**, you should feel the shoulder blades and the muscles around them contracting and squeezing together. This movement in the water will work the major muscle groups in the chest and back.

Repeat 10 times.

Again, check in with how you feel. Float around a little. Sore? Taxed? That's okay, enjoy the water for a little bit more, call it a win, and look forward to the next workout.

If you have a little gas left in the tank, do one more set.

The goal is three sets of 10 repetitions.

Finish where you started. Four laps the length of the pool, same instruction points on the work load. Heart rate slightly elevated, but not too much. After being sick and sedentary, this will feel challenging.

In the beginning, it felt like my heart was going to burst through my chest. My heart was pumping so hard, I could clearly hear the thumping. Initially, I was pushing too hard. I underestimated how physically beat down I was. Find your sweet spot and build slow and steady. This workout is laying the foundation of strength to build on, so execute it earnestly and consistently.

The goal, after at least two weeks depending on your starting condition, is to add a lap each session (one lap added to the warm-up and one lap added to the finishing cardio laps) and execute three sets of lower and upper body work. You'll get stronger; I did, but it will take time.

Record your work, how you feel before and after, physically, emotionally, and psychologically. You will see progress. Never underestimate the power of consistency, and do not get discouraged. It was not always easy to keep spirits positive, but it is possible, and it is better for your long-term health to do so. And hanging in the negative space is not helpful.

I still have my swim journals. I did this workout for six weeks before I started adding more. 4 laps, 2 sets legs, 2 sets upper body finish 2 laps. That was all I could manage initially. And I had to be very careful and you should too getting in and out of the pool. The water gives buoyancy, so I was much more stable walking in water than on land at first. Don't get out of the water to land with a false sense of stability. Make sure to have your stability under you coming out of the water before you start walking to your towel, the locker room, etc.

Hold the hand rails getting in and out of the pool. Just take it slow and know over time you will get stronger. Six weeks is a reasonable time frame to start expecting to feel stronger. Your body will adapt to the new demands you are placing on it. As it adapts, it is time to add new demands. After a couple weeks, I decided to teach myself how to swim.

You may want to stay with aqua exercises without adding the learning to swim component. I recommend learning to swim. Why not? What else do you have to do? And you shouldn't give up the aqua strength training while adding in some swimming challenges. By the way, teaching yourself to swim will take a lot of mental focus. Trust me, the brain power is better spent there than focused on the disease.

Okay good, so you're on the swim journey. Sweet! In the warm-up and ending laps associated with the workout I assigned, turn two of those walking/jogging laps into a swim lap. It doesn't have to be pretty, in fact it probably won't be, and it won't be easy.

So just do it and pay attention to how you move. From there you grow. It took me two years until I was proficient. During my evolution in the water, I learned most swimmers are very friendly, love to swim, and really love to help others learn. If someone at your facility is offering you tips, take them! One day you will return the favor.

Also, the best resource I found was the "Go Swim" channel on YouTube. Watch the videos, then slowly and diligently implement the movement in the water. Pick one stroke to learn first. I started with the breast stroke. That just seems to come more naturally to me than freestyle, although the opposite is true for many others.

Great! Here you are six weeks into your water progress, and you've decided to take the challenge to teach yourself to swim. Keep going. This is a life-long process, baby steps to who knows where. Provided you're working in a judicious, slightly challenging, and progressive manner, you will be unstoppable.

I started as a total novice in the water in December 2011. I worked out 2-3 times a week in the water while teaching myself to swim.

By May 2012, I decided I was strong enough to add in land exercises. The time frame is a year after the first wake up unable to walk, and six months after I started the water exercise program. When you add in land exercises depends on your own status, primarily judging your overall stability. You may be ready right now.

Land Workout

This workout, complete with basic stretching, will take 40 minutes.

First, walk outside for 20 minutes.

Outside is important (just watch out for ticks! LOL). Get fresh air, breathe deeply. Clear your mind. Walking can be meditative. Take this time to think about your day, count your blessings, be grateful for your family, and appreciate the beauty of the world.

Do this year-round; weather is no excuse to not get out. Below is a list of essential gear:

1) Baseball cap and sunglasses.

2) Good sneakers for three seasons, no flip-flops for summer, no exceptions. For winter, a good pair of boots with sturdy rubber soles. Allow for thick warm socks, make sure to buy appropriately sized boots.

3) Umbrella and/or raincoat. A good cap and raincoat are enough for me, but if you hate being wet, get the umbrella so the rain will not present a reason not to walk.

4) Fuzzy fun ear muffs, a special walking scarf, and gloves.

* * *

Now you're back from your walk, your heart is pumping, and your blood is oxygenated. Time for your strengthening exercises. The 4 exercise circuit of compound exercises will train all your major muscle groups and in turn will support your joints.

Each exercise is performed for 40 seconds with a 20-second break between. Move to the next exercise. Repeat 4 times. Total time is 16 minutes.

1) Squat: 40 seconds/break 20 seconds

2) Push-ups: 40 seconds/break 20 seconds

3) Sit-ups: 40 seconds/break 20 seconds

4) Back extensions: 40 seconds/break 20 seconds

Total time so far: 36 minutes.

4 minutes to stretch.

Hold each stretch for 30 seconds, breathing deeply, in the nose and out the mouth.

1) Chest opener: Stand in a doorway, place hands on door frame, hands at shoulder level, lean forward.

2) Back opener: Still in doorway, hold door frame with finger tips, lean back. Breathing deeply, feel shoulder blades opening and base of neck relaxing.

3) Posterior chain release: Stand feet shoulder-width apart. Reach arms to ceiling, with a deep breath, reach ALL the way up to the ceiling, even through the fingers. With a big exhale, fall forward to touch the toes. Take three big breaths, falling deep into the stretch. Roll up slowly, stacking one vertebrae on top of the other.

4) Lateral side stretch: Big breath, reach up and over with right hand leaning over to left side. Three big breaths. With the last exhale, rise to neutral, big breath in, up and over with left hand bending to the right side. Three big breaths. Last exhale rise to neutral. And you're off to your great day!

MAKE FRIENDS WITH PAIN

Over the years I have gotten stronger and stronger. From getting in the water December 2011 to today, physically, I am a different person. My capacities are greater, and my limitations have been isolated to my left hip. I lift weights regularly, and I keep my cardiovascular system healthy by swimming. I still can't run, at least not without paying for it. My left hip has stabilized, and being strong helps that joint enormously, but it is a damaged joint that I have to work around and sometimes baby.

Thinking back, the best I can remember is a "spider bite" I had on the back of my left knee. The main reason I remember the bite is that it was the size of a quarter, extremely red and gnarly, and I was worried it would show through my pantyhose and ruin the look of the dress I was planning to wear for our rehearsal dinner. That would have been late summer 2009. I don't remember feeling sick, at least not in any significantly memorable way. I simply treated the bite with topical medicine, hoping to avoid scarring, but it never seemed like cause to go to a doctor. I kept track of the bite, mainly motivated by vanity, and it was gone by September, in time for our wedding.

I hadn't thought of the bite again until June 2017, when I read an article summarizing a recent medical publication. The publication discussed cases of people who had gone to a doctor for a severe spider bite, were tested for Lyme just in case (like I said, the Northeast is getting WAY more vigilant), and the tests were positive. The main hypothesis the article highlighted was that sometimes tick bites could present more like a spider bite, rather than the bulls-eye rash. The aim of the article was to educate and encourage people to go to the doctor and get tested for Lyme if they have what might normally be passed off as a "spider bite." Better safe than sorry.

I thought, hmmm, maybe; but I'll never know for certain. Still, chances are pretty good that the "spider" bite I had in late summer 2009 was the bite that infected me. I've never had a bite, or a reaction to a bite like that before or since. So, if I were betting the odds, I say I probably had Lyme tooling around in my body for about two years before it really made itself known. The delay in treatment set me up with two separate, but still Lyme-related problems: Lyme arthritis, specifically in my left hip, and a propensity toward flare-ups.

Lyme arthritis is just arthritis. Sometimes it completely alleviates, but the longer the initial infection remains untreated, the less alleviation the originally attacked joint will enjoy. In that case it is just an arthritic joint; no more, no less. However, after initial Lyme treatment, the arthritis should not further progress, nor will it become bilateral or multi joint the way, for example, an autoimmune disease would.

My story and everything I have learned from the experience that I'm sharing with you is with the single aim to help you to help yourself. I want you to give yourself the opportunity to feel your best by arming your body with a nutrient-dense, low-sugar diet while bolstering your body through exercise. My hope is that my Lyme hacks enable you to feel better than you normally do, to the point that dealing with chronic Lyme 95% of the time is almost a nonissue. I'd take that as a win. But the truth is, sometimes you are going to have real setbacks. I still do.

Crushing generalized joint pain, demoralizing exhaustion, full-body weakness, and mental fog often accompanied by mood destabilization seem to be the most common ailments of post treatment Lyme. If, like me, you had a delay in treatment, you probably experienced these symptoms recurring over the years. My wish for you is that by taking care of your body and making it the lean, feisty machine it is designed to be, you can whittle flare-ups down to once or twice per year. That is where I currently am. As time has gone on and I keep up with my smart eating and diligent exercise, the period between flare-ups continues to lengthen, though the intensity has not lessened.

In my experience, the symptoms express concurrently and quickly, without exception. I haven't been able to establish a clear pattern in relation to time of year or stress, for example, as contributing factors to flare-ups. My diet and exercise are remarkably consistent as variations do have consequences, so that doesn't seem like a flare-up variable. Certain things I simply haven't been able to pin down.

As I grew in to my new body, accepting the new rules Lyme had laid out for me, I kept on the path to getting stronger and eating the best I possibly could. By May 2012, I was judiciously adding land exercises to my routine. Slowly but surely, I was expanding my abilities. I was doing the exact workout I included above.

Twice a week I'd go to the pool, I walked every morning, and two other days I did not have on the schedule to go to the pool, I did the resistance sequence, body weight only. The year of 2012 that was all I did. As I grew stronger, I increased the frequency, not intensity (meaning I stayed at body weight and increased repetitions, my joints weren't yet ready for heavy loads), of the land work, and kept at it in the pool. By the end of 2012 I was getting proficient at swimming.

Early spring 2013, I received an email from SUNY New Paltz stating that students from the collegiate swim team were offering free swim lessons to alumni. I jumped on the opportunity. The students were great, helped me improve my technique, and gave me mega props for how well I swam without ever having had a formal lesson. The acknowledgment of a job well done from people whose expertise far outweighed mine gave me a sense of satisfaction and pride.

Exercise and good food were paying dividends. But still, at a relatively young age, I had arthritis in my left hip, and at least quarterly I was having ass-kicking flare-ups. Even though I had come far over the 2 years, I still felt like I was fighting an uphill battle.

So, spring 2013, I took some downtime. I used a week of vacation for a staycation. I simply wanted to reflect on how far I'd come, where I was stuck, where I'd like to see improvements, and finally determine what constituted realistic expectations. During quiet reflection, I admitted what I think I had already known but had not fully realized. The experience of getting Lyme, being crippled—albeit THANKFULY temporally—and having to take real control over my health, had changed me. Although I loved my career and the overall structure of my life, it was clear that it was time to make a change. I decided to end my career in real estate and finance and start over in the field of fitness and nutrition. Over the course of 2013 I slowly made the transition while taking classes and obtaining the proper certifications.

The more I learned, the more I fine-tuned my workout regimen, and the harder I pushed my physical limits. By 2014, I was regularly lifting progressively heavier weights and still eating by the principles I laid out in this work, just in larger portions. My hip was a hinderance, but I'd learned to work with the limitation and pain.

Through the year 2014, I felt well most of the time, but I still felt the push and pull of the disease. The stronger and more physically self-possessed I became, the weaker it felt like the disease was becoming, but still Lyme frequently felt like a pushy monster that wanted to take over and have a party in my body. I know this sounds strange. It certainly feels odd writing this down, but I often felt like the disease was waiting, lurking, and searching for a sign of weakness so that it may again take over in my body. In a peculiar way, I began to respect its will to live; I just didn't like that it was trying to do it in my body.

Between the years 2014 and 2016 I had an average of two flare-ups per year. The frequency of the flare-ups was cut in half, which was tolerable, but the flare-ups themselves were still debilitating and time consuming.

But by the end of 2016 toward 2017, I noticed something. Nary a flare-up, nor a joint complaint outside of the standard hip trouble. I looked back over 2016 and realized I had only one flare-up, in March. Nine months had passed, and nothing! What a treat!

Maybe I was done, maybe I had gotten my health so dialed in that the disease was too weak to put up any sort of a legitimate fight, maybe I finally kicked it. I didn't know and didn't want to overthink it. I was scheduled to go for my biannual physical in February 2017 anyway, so I decided I address the update with my doctor then.

The blood test showed the usual, 8 of the 14 Lyme bands showed as reactive. The conversation was the same as usual, the infection isn't technically active, but you still have activity in your body, keep up the good work, and hopefully, you'll stay feeling good. It's always some version of that. The doctors are doing the best they can, but there still is a fair amount of mystery when dealing with Lyme.

I just kept on my trajectory of growing my new career and keeping myself in tip-top shape. Then, WHAM! In early August 2017 my wrists started to hurt. Both, simultaneously, equally and suddenly, and then my lower back, which had never happened before. And then, it quickly moved into my hips, knees, shoulders, ankles, everything but my neck. DONE! What the hell!? I was secretly hoping, more than hoping, secretly assuming, I was done with this, even though my doctor told me to keep my expectations realistic.

Well, she was back, and back with a vengeance. I paid dearly for the gift of the flare-up-free year I had enjoyed. Jaw-clenching pain, and close to total immobility was the price. By the second week in August I was toast, ankle to wrist.

Again, we were living downstairs because I couldn't do the stairs. My ankles were so swollen that I didn't have enough mobility to step up and down the stairs. This was by far the worst flare-up. During that same week the fatigue came so powerfully, I wouldn't have believed it unless I lived it myself.

I had family obligations the week of the 13th. My mother had flown in from Florida (yes, all New Yorkers do move to Florida after age 65) for a couple of bridal and baby shower celebrations. I was doing the absolute bare minimum possible, and even that was taking everything out of me. By the end of that week I was scarcely functional.

I was a wet blanket sitting in the background during the joyous celebrations for my nieces. I didn't want to attract attention to my downgraded health and away from my nieces, so my sisters helped me get in a tolerable position on a fluffily covered outdoor lounger, and there I stayed.

I'm hyper by personality, so extended friends and family where curious, but we all, sisters and Mom, agreed to pass off my out-of-character behavior as a result of being exhausted from a long week of teaching fitness classes. A true enough statement, it was a polite deflection back to the girls.

Bob picked me up from the party on Saturday. I had been carpooling and getting rides most of that week because I was in too much pain to drive, and I promptly fell asleep in the car. I vaguely remember getting home. From there I went to sleep, until Monday morning. I of course stirred here and there, but I can safely say I slept for nearly 30 hours.

The sleep helped, but I was still really hurting. After sleep-resting since some time Saturday, when I woke Monday, I wiggled a little under the covers. The tiny bit of resistance from the blankets sent waves of pain from every joint so intensely, it occurred to me that suicide was a viable option. I flopped my head toward Bob's side of the bed and mumbled, "Maybe I should just kill myself, kind of wrap up this whole nonsense."

This was the first, and only, time I contemplated suicide as a result of dealing with Lyme. I proposed the pro-suicide argument casually and calculatingly. Though I was laying the case from a flawed premise, I thought I made a viable argument. I felt beat, and I didn't want to muster up any more will or energy to fight. Suicide seemed like a viable option.

Of course, Bob simply said, "Nope."

That was it. Sometimes he's a man of few words. He did however stay next to me in bed for a little extra time that morning. I could tell he was waiting for me to work out my flawed thinking. Though he was quiet, his presence was strong. We laid in bed in silence for a little longer, then Bob got up and started helping me get up. He ran through the morning routine and was out the door to work.

The house was quiet and still, and I was alone. I had to get dreadfully honest with myself. Most of the time, 90-95% of the time, I was generally so much better, and 100% different from whence all this started. I was stronger, had adopted a new perspective on life, but maybe along this wonderful journey, I had gotten a little cocky.

I had learned and applied valuable lessons to my life, but with that growth came some hubris. I had let myself think I had this whole business under my control, and this flare up was back to let me know that was not the truth. Besides being sick, I was deflated, knocked down a peg.

I reminded myself how far I'd come, and that I knew how to muster up emotional and physical fortitude, and that it was time again to do so. I just needed to get some fresh air, clear my mind. That Monday, August 21st, 2017, a solar eclipse was predicted. That unique phenomenon gave me a little more motivation to get up and out for an afternoon "hike".

I went to the stunning Spring Farm Trail on Mohonk Mountain, which is part of the Shawangunk Mountain range here in the Hudson Valley. I walked as diligently as I could. Each step was painful, with a funky gait. During my mini trek, I learned and remembered a couple of things. Maybe it's more accurate to state I synthesized some things I knew but hadn't integrated yet.

First, I needed to reset the gratitude lesson I learned early on. I had come so far that I had forgotten the sheer joy of the gift of being ambulatory. I have never been as debilitated as I first was, which is something I should not allow myself to forget or become complacent about. I decided that although I wanted to keep progressing in my fitness levels, it was imperative to find a mindset that enabled me to push to my limits but still be genuinely grateful for the gains I had made.

The progress I had made over the years pushed me to want more, and more. Which in and of itself is a fine thing, but that mindset was pulling me away from the initial trill of regaining my health and set me up for a huge emotional crash when I got knocked back on my ass. I needed to be better at striving with humility as a guide, instead of the arrogance that had crept in the mental side door and had become the driver.

Second, I realized it was time for me to make friends with pain and make peace with the disease. Over the course of this process the pain sometimes had been so intense that I developed a fear of it. I don't know how, for so many years, I missed this fact, but I did. Physical pain is no picnic, but it is far more tolerable if you can detach from it emotionally. It took some time, but as I began to look at pain as a tool, I became less afraid, and from there a lot of the emotions associated with pain evaporated. Pain is just a warning system whose primary purpose is self-preservation. In a way, pain is a gift. Being brave and facing pain dispassionately while trying to attend to the physical ailment the pain is alerting is a difficult balance to achieve and maintain, but it is a worthy and liberating task.

The raw calculating logic of pain detachment also showed me that I was, in an odd way, attached to the disease. I didn't like it, we weren't friends, but in a way, it was a part of who I was, by always fighting it I was, in a way, empowering it. I decided on that slow walk in the woods to have a chat with the disease. I know this sounds totally crazy, but it's true.

First, I made sure I was out of ear shot from any other hikers. Then, I said out loud, "Fine, its obvious you're not going anywhere—at least for the time being, but if you want to live here, you have to fucking cooperate."—"I'm in charge here, and this is my body, not yours-, if I have to I will share, but on my terms—you don't get to keep taking over like this." A simple enough claim, but it helped clarify my target.

It reminded me to keep up the fight, for me, for my long-term mental and physical health. The fight shouldn't be for me tangled up with and somewhat defined by the disease. It's not Jen powering through despite Lyme, it's Jen powering through. The mind set change was subtle but significant.

FOOD MOVEMENT MIND

So, there you have it. My story. The loss and regain of health has shaped and reshaped me in a variety of ways. I hope my story resonates with you and lets you know I'm right there with you, as are a lot of people. We're all friends in our triumphs and backslides.

Take my recommendations, make them your own, improve upon them, and let us all know how we can keep tweaking our daily habits, so we can maximize every day.

Good food, smartly executed exercise, and sound strong mind are what I hope I offered in this work.

Happy healing! Lyme be damned!